Promoting Healthy Eating Habits

Edet Amos

INTRODUCTION:

Promoting healthy eating habits is a critical
endeavour in today's society, where the
prevalence of diet-related health issues such as
obesity, heart disease, and diabetes continues to
rise. This multifaceted approach focuses on
encouraging individuals and communities to
make informed choices that prioritise nutrition
and overall well-being. By fostering an
environment that supports and advocates for
healthier food choices, we can enhance the
quality of life, reduce the burden on healthcare
systems, and promote a sustainable future.

Healthy eating habits encompass more than just
what goes on one's plate; they are a reflection of
cultural, social, economic, and psychological
factors. This introduction explores the
significance of promoting healthy eating habits
and delves into the various aspects that influence
our dietary choices. It highlights the importance

of education, access to nutritious options, and the role of policy initiatives in shaping our food environment. Ultimately, the promotion of healthy eating habits is a holistic approach that not only impacts individuals but also has broader implications for public health, environmental sustainability, and societal well-being.

TABLE OF CONTENTS

Topic :1 "The Impact of Nutrition Education" in promoting healthier eating habits:

Nutrition education is a fundamental component of efforts to improve dietary choices and overall health. It encompasses a wide range of strategies and initiatives aimed at increasing individuals' knowledge and understanding of nutrition, food choices, and their impact on health. Here's a more detailed exploration of this important aspect of promoting healthy eating habits:

School-Based Nutrition Education: Nutrition education often begins in schools, where students are taught about the importance of a balanced diet, food groups, portion control, and the nutritional value of different foods. Schools may incorporate nutrition into their curriculum, offer cooking classes, or maintain partnerships with organisations that provide nutrition education.

Community-Based Programs: Beyond schools, community-based programs play a vital role in nutrition education. These initiatives can include workshops, cooking demonstrations, and informational sessions held in community centres, libraries, or healthcare facilities. They target diverse audiences, including adults, parents, and senior citizens.

Online Resources: In the digital age, online resources have become increasingly important for nutrition education. Websites, apps, and social media platforms provide easy access to a wealth of information about healthy eating, recipes, meal planning, and dietary guidelines. These resources can reach a wide audience and empower individuals to make informed choices.

Healthcare Professionals: Registered dietitians and healthcare professionals are valuable sources of nutrition education. They work with patients to create personalised dietary plans, offer guidance on managing medical conditions through diet, and provide ongoing support and education.

Public Awareness Campaigns: Governments and non-profit organisations often run public awareness campaigns to promote healthy eating habits. These campaigns use various media channels to disseminate messages about the benefits of healthy eating, the risks of unhealthy diets, and practical tips for making better food

Topic:2 "Healthy Eating in Childhood":

Healthy eating habits established during childhood are pivotal for a lifetime of good health and well-being. The early years of life are a critical period for growth and development, making it essential to provide children with the right nutrients and dietary patterns. Here's a more detailed exploration of this important aspect of promoting healthy eating habits in childhood:

Nutritional Needs in Childhood: Children have unique nutritional needs due to their rapid growth and development. These needs include essential nutrients like vitamins, minerals, protein, and healthy fats. A balanced diet is crucial to support their physical and cognitive development.

Impact on Growth: Proper nutrition in childhood directly influences physical growth. Nutrients like calcium, vitamin D, and protein are vital for bone development, while iron is necessary for cognitive development. Poor nutrition during this period can lead to growth stunting or developmental delays.

Establishing Taste Preferences: Childhood is when taste preferences are formed. Introducing a variety of nutritious foods at an early age can help children develop a preference for healthier options. It's an opportunity to cultivate a lifelong love for fruits, vegetables, and whole grains.

Preventing Childhood Obesity: Healthy eating habits play a significant role in preventing childhood obesity, which has become a global health concern. Educating children about balanced nutrition and portion control can help reduce the risk of obesity-related health issues, such as diabetes and heart disease.

Family and Environmental Influences: The family and home environment have a substantial impact on children's eating habits. Parents and caregivers can serve as role models by demonstrating healthy eating behaviours and creating a supportive food environment at home.

School Nutrition Programs: School lunch programs and policies can influence what children eat during the school day. Initiatives to improve the nutritional quality of school meals and provide nutrition education in schools are critical for promoting healthy eating in childhood.

Media and Advertising: Media, including television and online platforms, can significantly influence children's food choices. The marketing of unhealthy foods to children is a concern, highlighting the importance of regulating advertising and promoting media literacy among young consumers.

Food Accessibility: Access to healthy foods is essential. In some areas, known as food deserts, access to fresh produce and nutritious options may be limited. Addressing food access disparities is crucial for ensuring all children have the opportunity to eat healthily.

Behavioural Strategies: Behavioural strategies, such as positive reinforcement, role modelling, and involving children in meal planning and preparation, can be effective in encouraging healthy eating habits.

Health Education in Schools: Incorporating nutrition education into school curricula can empower children with the knowledge and skills needed to make healthier food choices independently.

Topic:3 "Nutrition Labels and Food Choices":

Nutrition labels play a crucial role in helping consumers make informed choices about the foods they purchase and consume. These labels provide detailed information about the nutritional content of products, serving sizes, and ingredients. Here's a more detailed exploration of the impact of nutrition labels on food choices and overall health:

Understanding Nutrition Labels: Nutrition labels typically include information on calories, macronutrients (such as fats, carbohydrates, and proteins), micronutrients (such as vitamins and minerals), and other relevant details like serving sizes and daily recommended values. Understanding these labels is essential for consumers to assess the nutritional quality of foods accurately.

Promoting Informed Choices: Nutrition labels empower consumers to make informed decisions about the foods they buy. They can compare products, assess their nutritional value, and choose options that align with their dietary preferences and health goals.

Calorie Awareness: Calorie information on nutrition labels helps individuals manage their calorie intake, which is crucial for weight management and overall health. Knowing the number of calories in a serving helps consumers control portion sizes and make choices that fit their daily energy needs.

Sugar, Salt, and Fat Content: Nutrition labels highlight the content of added sugars, sodium (salt), and various types of fats, including saturated and trans fats. High consumption of these elements is linked to health issues such as obesity, heart disease, and hypertension. Nutrition labels enable consumers to identify products with excessive amounts of these ingredients.

Serving Sizes: Nutrition labels specify serving sizes, which are essential for accurate nutritional assessment. Consumers can gauge whether they are consuming an appropriate portion and how many servings are in a package.

Comparing Products: Nutrition labels make it easier to compare similar products and select the one with better nutritional value. Consumers can look for lower levels of saturated fat, sugar, and sodium and higher levels of beneficial nutrients like fibre and vitamins.

Special Dietary Needs: Nutrition labels can be particularly valuable for individuals with specific dietary requirements, such as those with food allergies or intolerances. Clear labelling of allergens helps them avoid potential health risks.

Health Claims and Labels: Some products carry health claims or labels like "low-fat," "organic," or "gluten-free." Understanding the meaning of these claims is essential for consumers seeking products that align with their health and lifestyle preferences.

Nutrition Education: Nutrition labels also serve as a tool for nutrition education. They can help individuals become more knowledgeable about the nutritional content of various foods and ingredients, ultimately promoting better food choices.

Policy Impact: Government regulations and policies play a role in shaping nutrition labels and their format. Policy changes, such as requiring added sugar labelling or updating serving sizes to reflect real-world consumption, can have a significant impact on consumer choices.

Topic :4 "Cultural Influences on Diet" and how cultural backgrounds and traditions affect eating habits:

Diversity of Cultural Influences: Cultural influences on diet are incredibly diverse, as they are shaped by historical, geographical, and social factors. Different cultures have distinct food traditions, cooking methods, and dietary preferences that reflect their unique heritage and values.

Traditional Diets: Many cultures have traditional diets that are often rich in locally sourced ingredients. These diets can be quite healthy, emphasising fresh fruits and vegetables, lean proteins, and whole grains. Examples include the Mediterranean diet, Japanese diet, and traditional diets of Indigenous peoples.

Cultural Significance of Food: Food often holds cultural significance beyond mere sustenance. It can play a central role in rituals, celebrations, and social gatherings. Understanding the cultural importance of certain foods can shed light on why they are consumed and in what contexts.

Food Preparation and Cooking Techniques: Cultural influences extend to food preparation and cooking techniques. The way food is cooked, seasoned, and presented can vary widely between cultures. For instance, stir-frying in Asian cuisines, slow cooking in Mediterranean cuisines, and the use of spices in Indian cuisine are all distinctive culinary traditions.

Dietary Restrictions: Some cultural or religious practices may lead to dietary restrictions. For example, in Islam, adherents observe halal dietary laws, which influence the types of foods and preparation methods allowed. Similarly, Hinduism and Buddhism have vegetarian traditions.

Migration and Acculturation: As people migrate and settle in new regions, their dietary habits may evolve due to exposure to different foods and culinary practices. This process of acculturation can lead to a blending of dietary traditions and the adoption of new foods.

Health Implications: Cultural dietary patterns can have varying health implications. While some traditional diets are associated with lower rates of chronic diseases, others may contribute to health issues when combined with modern, sedentary lifestyles.

Promoting Healthy Eating within Cultural Context: Encouraging healthier eating habits within cultural contexts can be complex. It often involves respecting cultural traditions while finding ways to adapt or modify certain aspects of the diet to improve overall health.

Community-Based Approaches: Community-based initiatives can be effective in promoting healthier eating habits within cultural communities. These programs involve community members in designing culturally relevant nutrition education and cooking classes.

Cultural Competence in Healthcare: Healthcare providers need to be culturally competent, understanding the dietary preferences and restrictions of their patients. This enables them to provide culturally sensitive dietary recommendations and improve health outcomes.

Food Equity and Cultural Diversity: Addressing food equity is essential to ensure that culturally diverse communities have access to fresh, culturally relevant ingredients. It involves reducing disparities in food access, affordability, and quality.

Globalisation and Fusion Cuisine: Globalisation has led to the fusion of culinary traditions, resulting in innovative and diverse cuisines. While fusion cuisine can be exciting, it also raises questions about preserving traditional dietary practices and cultural authenticity.

Topic :5 "The Role of Government Policies" in promoting healthy eating habits:

Regulation and Oversight: Government policies play a crucial role in regulating the food industry to ensure food safety, quality, and labelling accuracy. Regulatory agencies, such as the FDA in the United States, are responsible for enforcing these policies.

Nutrition Labelling: Government policies often mandate the inclusion of nutrition labels on packaged foods. These labels provide consumers with essential information about the nutritional content of products, including calorie counts, macronutrients, and daily recommended values.

Sugary Beverage Taxes: Some governments have implemented taxes on sugary beverages to reduce consumption and combat obesity and related health issues. These taxes aim to discourage the consumption of high-sugar, calorie-dense drinks.

School Nutrition Programs: Governments frequently establish and fund school nutrition programs to ensure that students have access to healthy meals. These programs may set nutritional standards for school lunches and snacks, promoting balanced diets among children.

Food Marketing and Advertising Regulations: Policies can govern the marketing and advertising practices of food companies, particularly concerning products targeted at children. Restrictions on advertising unhealthy foods to kids aim to reduce their exposure to persuasive marketing.

Food Assistance Programs: Government initiatives like food assistance programs (e.g., SNAP in the U.S.) help low-income individuals and families access nutritious foods. These programs promote food security and reduce the risk of hunger and malnutrition.

Menu Labelling in Restaurants: In some regions, governments require restaurants and food service establishments to provide calorie and nutrition information on menus. This empowers consumers to make informed choices when dining out.

Front-of-Package Labelling: Governments may establish guidelines for front-of-package labelling systems, making it easier for consumers to identify healthier food options. These systems often use symbols, colours, or logos to indicate the nutritional quality of products.

Food Subsidies and Farm Policies: Agricultural and farm policies can influence the production and pricing of different food types. Subsidies that support the production of fruits and vegetables, for example, can make these healthy foods more affordable.

Food Safety Regulations: Ensuring the safety of the food supply is a primary responsibility of governments. Regulations related to food processing, storage, and transportation are in place to prevent foodborne illnesses.

Promotion of Healthier Food Environments: Some governments work to create environments that encourage healthy eating. This may involve zoning laws that limit the density of fast-food restaurants in certain areas or incentives for food retailers to establish stores in underserved communities.

Research and Public Health Initiatives: Governments often fund research on nutrition and public health. The results of this research inform policy decisions and public health campaigns aimed at promoting healthier eating habits.

International Agreements: International organisations and agreements, such as the World Health Organization (WHO) and Codex Alimentarius, set global standards and guidelines for food safety and nutrition, influencing national policies.

Topic :6 "Nutrition in the Workplace" and explore strategies for promoting healthy eating habits in the workplace:

Workplace Wellness Programs: Many organisations implement workplace wellness programs to encourage healthier lifestyles among employees. These programs often include components related to nutrition, such as nutrition education sessions, cooking classes, and access to healthy snacks.

Healthy Cafeteria and Vending Options: Employers can influence employees' eating habits by providing healthy food options in workplace cafeterias and vending machines. This can include offering a variety of fresh fruits, vegetables, lean proteins, and whole grains.

Nutrition Labelling: Clear nutrition labelling in workplace food service areas can help employees make informed choices about their meals. Labels that provide information on calorie counts, ingredients, and allergens are valuable.

Nutrition Education: Hosting nutrition workshops or seminars in the workplace can educate employees about the importance of balanced nutrition, portion control, and making healthy food choices. Nutritionists or registered dietitians can be invited to provide expert guidance.

Healthy Snack Policies: Encouraging the availability of healthy snacks in the workplace can discourage the consumption of less nutritious options. Employers can stock break rooms and vending machines with items like fresh fruit, nuts, and yoghurt.

Meal Planning and Cooking Classes: Offering cooking classes or meal planning workshops can empower employees to prepare healthier meals at home. Teaching practical cooking skills and providing recipes can make healthy eating more accessible.

Nutrition Challenges and Incentives: Some workplaces organise nutrition challenges or competitions to motivate employees to adopt healthier eating habits. Providing incentives, such as rewards or recognition, can boost participation.

Supportive Food Policies: Employers can establish policies that promote a culture of healthy eating. This might include discouraging the consumption of unhealthy foods at meetings or events and providing guidelines for catered meals.

Access to Clean Water: Access to clean drinking water in the workplace is essential for overall health. Encouraging employees to stay hydrated by providing water stations or reusable water bottles can support their well-being.

Physical Activity Integration: Combining nutrition initiatives with physical activity programs can create a holistic approach to employee well-being. Activities like walking meetings or on-site fitness facilities can complement healthy eating habits.

Flexible Meal Breaks: Allowing employees adequate time for meal breaks enables them to make healthier meal choices. Rushed or skipped meals are more likely to lead to unhealthy food choices.

Wellness Challenges: Workplace wellness challenges that incorporate healthy eating components, such as tracking fruit and vegetable consumption or reducing sugar intake, can engage employees and foster a sense of community.

Health Screening and Assessments: Offering health screenings and assessments can help employees understand their nutritional needs and identify areas for improvement.

Supportive Work Environment: Creating a supportive work environment for healthy eating includes fostering a workplace culture that values and priorities employee health. Support from leadership and peers can be motivating.

Feedback and Evaluation: Regularly seeking feedback from employees about workplace nutrition initiatives allows for adjustments and improvements over time. Evaluating the effectiveness of these programs can guide future efforts.

Topic :7 "Community-Based Nutrition Programs" and explore how these initiatives can effectively promote healthy eating habits within communities:

Targeted Community Outreach: Community-based nutrition programs often begin with targeted outreach efforts. They aim to identify the specific nutritional needs and challenges within a community, taking into account factors like demographics, cultural diversity, and socioeconomic status.

Nutrition Education: Central to these programs is nutrition education. This involves teaching community members about the basics of balanced nutrition, understanding food labels, portion control, and making healthier food choices. Nutrition education can be delivered through workshops, classes, or community events.

Culturally Tailored Initiatives: Recognizing the cultural diversity within communities, these programs often tailor their approach to align with local traditions and dietary preferences. Culturally sensitive materials and strategies can enhance engagement and relevance.

Cooking Classes and Demonstrations: Practical cooking classes and cooking demonstrations are effective tools for teaching individuals how to prepare nutritious meals. These hands-on experiences can improve cooking skills and confidence in making healthy choices.

Access to Healthy Foods: Addressing food access disparities is a key component of community-based nutrition programs. This may involve initiatives to increase the availability of fresh fruits and vegetables in underserved areas, supporting farmers' markets, or establishing community gardens.

Community Gardens: Community gardens provide not only a source of fresh produce but also a sense of community and empowerment. These initiatives enable residents to grow their own fruits and vegetables, fostering a deeper connection to healthy foods.

Policy Advocacy: Some community-based programs engage in advocacy efforts to influence local policies related to food access, marketing of unhealthy foods, and school nutrition. Policy changes can have a lasting impact on the community's food environment.

Collaboration with Local Organisations: Collaboration with local healthcare providers, schools, faith-based organisations, and community centres can extend the reach and impact of these programs. Partnering with existing community networks can enhance program effectiveness.

Involving Community Leaders: Engaging community leaders and influencers can help build trust and support for nutrition initiatives. These individuals can help promote healthy eating as a community value.

Behavioural Change Strategies: Behavior change theories and strategies, such as social support networks and goal setting, are often integrated into community-based nutrition programs to help individuals adopt and maintain healthier eating habits.

Measurement and Evaluation: Evaluating the impact of these programs is crucial. This involves tracking changes in dietary behaviours, food access, and health outcomes within the community to assess program effectiveness.

Long-Term Sustainability: Ensuring the long-term sustainability of community-based nutrition programs is essential. This may involve training community members to become program leaders and advocates, securing funding, and fostering a sense of ownership within the community.

Youth and School Involvement: Engaging youth in nutrition programs can have a ripple effect, as they often influence their families' dietary choices. School-based initiatives, nutrition education in schools, and after-school programs can all contribute to healthier eating habits among young community members.

Promotion of Local Food Systems: Encouraging the support of local food systems and businesses can benefit both the community's economy and access to fresh, locally sourced foods.

Topic :8 "Online Resources for Healthy Eating" and how websites, apps, and social media platforms contribute to promoting healthier eating habits:

Nutritional Information and Guidance: Online resources provide a wealth of information about nutrition, dietary guidelines, and healthy eating tips. Websites and apps often feature articles, blogs, and interactive tools that help individuals understand the nutritional content of foods and make informed choices.

Meal Planning and Tracking: Many online platforms offer meal planning tools and tracking apps that enable users to set dietary goals, plan balanced meals, and monitor their daily intake of calories, macronutrients, and micronutrients. These tools can enhance accountability and support healthier eating habits.

Recipe Databases: Online recipe databases and cooking websites are abundant. These platforms offer a wide range of healthy recipes that cater to various dietary preferences and restrictions. Users can search for recipes based on specific ingredients, cuisines, or dietary goals.

Mobile Apps for Healthy Eating: Mobile apps dedicated to healthy eating provide on-the-go access to nutrition information, recipe ideas, and meal tracking. Some apps offer personalised recommendations based on individual dietary needs and health goals.

Social Media Communities: Social media platforms like Instagram, Pinterest, and YouTube are hubs for sharing food inspiration and healthy eating tips. Many influencers, chefs, and nutritionists use these platforms to share visually appealing, nutritious meal ideas.

Online Cooking Classes: Virtual cooking classes and tutorials are available on platforms like YouTube and specialised cooking websites. These resources empower users to learn new cooking skills and experiment with healthier recipes from the comfort of their homes.

Food Blogs and Vlogs: Food bloggers and vloggers often focus on healthy eating, sharing their personal journeys, recipes, and lifestyle tips related to nutrition. These relatable voices can inspire and motivate individuals to adopt healthier habits.

Health and Nutrition Apps: Mobile apps designed specifically for health and nutrition provide a range of features, such as meal tracking, calorie counting, and fitness integration. Some apps offer community support and expert advice.

Online Communities and Forums: Online forums and communities dedicated to healthy eating provide a space for individuals to connect, share experiences, and seek advice. These platforms foster a sense of community and accountability.

Nutrition Analysis Tools: Online tools and calculators allow users to analyse the nutritional content of recipes they create or meals they consume. This can help individuals make adjustments to their diets to meet specific health goals.

Educational Websites: Educational websites from reputable sources, such as government health agencies and academic institutions, provide evidence-based information on nutrition and dietary recommendations. These resources help users separate reliable information from fads and misinformation.

Accessibility and Convenience: The convenience of online resources allows individuals to access nutrition information and healthy eating resources at any time, making it easier to make informed choices and plan nutritious meals.

Customised Dietary Plans: Some online platforms offer the option to create customised dietary plans based on individual preferences, dietary restrictions, and health conditions. These plans can help users meet their specific nutritional needs.

Topic :9 "Online Resources for Healthy Eating" and how websites, apps, and social media platforms contribute to promoting healthier eating habits:

Nutritional Information and Guidance: Online resources provide a wealth of information about nutrition, dietary guidelines, and healthy eating tips. Websites and apps often feature articles, blogs, and interactive tools that help individuals understand the nutritional content of foods and make informed choices.

Meal Planning and Tracking: Many online platforms offer meal planning tools and tracking apps that enable users to set dietary goals, plan balanced meals, and monitor their daily intake of calories, macronutrients, and micronutrients. These tools can enhance accountability and support healthier eating habits.

Recipe Databases: Online recipe databases and cooking websites are abundant. These platforms offer a wide range of healthy recipes that cater to various dietary preferences and restrictions. Users can search for recipes based on specific ingredients, cuisines, or dietary goals.

Mobile Apps for Healthy Eating: Mobile apps dedicated to healthy eating provide on-the-go access to nutrition information, recipe ideas, and meal tracking. Some apps offer personalised recommendations based on individual dietary needs and health goals.

Social Media Communities: Social media platforms like Instagram, Pinterest, and YouTube are hubs for sharing food inspiration and healthy eating tips. Many influencers, chefs, and nutritionists use these platforms to share visually appealing, nutritious meal ideas.

Online Cooking Classes: Virtual cooking classes and tutorials are available on platforms like YouTube and specialised cooking websites. These resources empower users to learn new cooking skills and experiment with healthier recipes from the comfort of their homes.

Food Blogs and Vlogs: Food bloggers and vloggers often focus on healthy eating, sharing their personal journeys, recipes, and lifestyle tips related to nutrition. These relatable voices can inspire and motivate individuals to adopt healthier habits.

Health and Nutrition Apps: Mobile apps designed specifically for health and nutrition provide a range of features, such as meal tracking, calorie counting, and fitness integration. Some apps offer community support and expert advice.

Online Communities and Forums: Online forums and communities dedicated to healthy eating provide a space for individuals to connect, share experiences, and seek advice. These platforms foster a sense of community and accountability.

Nutrition Analysis Tools: Online tools and calculators allow users to analyse the nutritional content of recipes they create or meals they consume. This can help individuals make adjustments to their diets to meet specific health goals.

Educational Websites: Educational websites from reputable sources, such as government health agencies and academic institutions, provide evidence-based information on nutrition and dietary recommendations. These resources help users separate reliable information from fads and misinformation.

Accessibility and Convenience: The convenience of online resources allows individuals to access nutrition information and healthy eating resources at any time, making it easier to make informed choices and plan nutritious meals.

Customised Dietary Plans: Some online platforms offer the option to create customised dietary plans based on individual preferences, dietary restrictions, and health conditions. These plans can help users meet their specific nutritional needs.

Topic :10   "The Influence of Marketing and Advertising on Dietary Choices" and explore the significant impact of marketing tactics on what people choose to eat:

Advertising and Food Choices: Advertising has a powerful influence on dietary choices. Food and beverage companies invest heavily in marketing strategies to promote their products and shape consumer preferences.

Targeted Marketing: Food advertisers often use targeted marketing to reach specific demographics, such as children, teenagers, or certain ethnic groups. Understanding their target audience allows advertisers to create persuasive campaigns tailored to individual preferences and interests.

Brand Recognition: Repetitive exposure to brand names and logos builds brand recognition. People are more likely to choose products they recognize and are familiar with, even if healthier alternatives are available.

Emotional Appeal: Many food advertisements evoke emotions, such as happiness, comfort, or indulgence, to create positive associations with their products. Emotional marketing can lead individuals to make food choices based on how they want to feel rather than their nutritional needs.

Portrayal of Health Claims: Some advertisements use health claims or labels like "low-fat," "natural," or "organic" to convey a sense of healthiness. These claims may not always align with the actual nutritional quality of the product.

Celebrity Endorsements: The use of celebrities and influencers in food advertising can be highly persuasive. People often admire and trust the endorsements of their favourite personalities, leading them to choose products associated with these figures.

Food Packaging and Presentation: The visual appeal of food packaging, such as colourful designs, appetising images, and attractive fonts, can make products more enticing. Packaging can influence perceptions of taste and quality.

Placement and Promotion: The strategic placement of products within stores and on menus can influence purchasing decisions. Products placed at eye level, near checkout counters, or on prominent menu boards are more likely to be chosen.

Price Promotions and Discounts: Discounts and special offers, such as "buy one, get one free" or meal deals, encourage bulk purchases and can sway consumers toward less nutritious options.

Online and Social Media Marketing: The rise of online marketing and social media has expanded the reach of food advertising. Influencers, bloggers, and sponsored content on platforms like Instagram and YouTube can subtly promote products to large audiences.

Interactive Marketing: Engaging consumers through interactive marketing campaigns, such as contests, games, or online quizzes, can create a sense of involvement and increase brand loyalty.

Food Desirability: Some advertisements create a perception of food as desirable or even addictive, leading individuals to over consume certain products. This is particularly concerning with regard to highly processed and sugary foods.

Regulatory Frameworks: Governments implement regulations and guidelines to restrict certain types of advertising, especially those targeting children, for unhealthy foods and beverages. However, enforcement and effectiveness of these regulations can vary.

Media Literacy: Promoting media literacy skills, especially among young people, can help individuals critically assess food advertisements and better understand their persuasive tactics.

Healthier Marketing Practices: Some food companies are adopting healthier marketing practices, such as promoting their healthier product lines or featuring nutrition information prominently in their advertising.

Topic :11 "Sustainable Food Choices" and explore the importance of sustainable eating habits for individuals and the planet:

Defining Sustainable Food Choices: Sustainable food choices involve selecting foods and dietary patterns that have a minimal negative impact on the environment, promote biodiversity, and support social and economic equity. Sustainable eating aims to balance human nutrition needs with environmental and ethical considerations.

Environmental Impact: Unsustainable food production practices, such as deforestation, overfishing, and excessive use of resources like water and fossil fuels, contribute to environmental degradation. Sustainable eating emphasises minimising these negative impacts.

Climate Change Mitigation: Agriculture and food production are significant contributors to greenhouse gas emissions. Sustainable food choices prioritise foods with lower carbon footprints, such as plant-based options, and advocate for reducing food waste to combat climate change.

Biodiversity Conservation: Industrial farming practices can lead to the loss of biodiversity, including the extinction of certain plant and animal species. Sustainable eating encourages the consumption of foods that support biodiversity conservation, such as heirloom varieties and sustainably sourced seafood.

Local and Seasonal Foods: Choosing locally grown and seasonal foods reduces the carbon footprint associated with food transportation and supports local economies. Sustainable eaters often prioritise foods produced closer to home.

Reducing Food Waste: Approximately one-third of the world's food is wasted. Sustainable food choices involve reducing food waste through mindful shopping, meal planning, and using leftovers creatively.

Plant-Based Diets: Plant-based diets, which emphasise fruits, vegetables, legumes, and whole grains while reducing or eliminating animal products, are considered more sustainable due to their lower environmental impact.

Ethical Considerations: Sustainable eating extends beyond environmental concerns to ethical considerations, such as fair labour practices, animal welfare, and supporting food systems that prioritise social equity.

Certifications and Labels: Certifications like "organic," "fair trade," and "Non-GMO" provide consumers with information about the sustainability and ethical practices associated with a product. Understanding these labels can guide sustainable food choices.

Reducing Highly Processed Foods: Highly processed foods often have a larger environmental footprint due to their resource-intensive production methods and packaging. Sustainable eating encourages the consumption of whole, minimally processed foods.

Educational Initiatives: Sustainable food choices are promoted through educational initiatives that raise awareness about the environmental and social impacts of different food choices. Schools, community organisations, and advocacy groups often play a role in these efforts.

Government Policies: Some governments are implementing policies and incentives to encourage sustainable food choices, such as subsidies for organic farming or restrictions on harmful agricultural practices.

Consumer Influence: Consumer demand for sustainable food choices can drive changes in the food industry. As more individuals choose sustainable products, food companies are more likely to adjust their practices to meet these preferences.

Food Systems Transformation: Achieving a truly sustainable food system requires systemic changes, including shifts in agricultural practices, supply chain management, and policy frameworks. Advocacy and collective action are essential in driving these changes.

Health and Sustainability: Sustainable eating can align with health goals, as many plant-based and whole foods are not only better for the environment but also beneficial for human health. This synergy supports long-term well-being.

Topic :12 "Childhood Nutrition and Healthy Eating Habits" and explore the critical role of early nutrition in shaping lifelong eating habits and overall health:

Early Development: Childhood nutrition is crucial because it directly impacts a child's growth, development, and overall health. Proper nutrition during this period supports the development of strong bones, healthy organs, and a robust immune system.

Formation of Habits: Childhood is a formative period when eating habits are established. The foods and dietary patterns children are exposed to during this time can shape their preferences and behaviours well into adulthood. Therefore, fostering healthy eating habits early is essential.

Nutrient Requirements: Children have unique nutrient requirements due to their growth and development. They need adequate amounts of essential nutrients like protein, calcium, iron, vitamins, and minerals. Meeting these needs is critical to ensure they thrive.

Balanced Diet: A balanced diet for children should include a variety of foods from different food groups, including fruits, vegetables, lean proteins, whole grains, and dairy or dairy alternatives. This variety provides the necessary nutrients for growth and health.

Mealtime Environment: Creating a positive mealtime environment is crucial. Family meals offer opportunities for children to learn about food, develop healthy eating habits, and enjoy social interactions. Mealtimes should be pleasant, without pressure or food-related stress.

Snacking Habits: Snacking is a part of most children's diets, and it's essential to promote healthy snack choices. Offering nutritious snacks like fruits, vegetables, and yoghourt can help children maintain energy levels between meals without excessive sugar or empty calories.

Hydration: Proper hydration is vital for children's health. Water should be the primary beverage, and sugary drinks should be limited. Teaching children to drink water when thirsty is a valuable habit.

Avoiding Excessive Sugars and Processed Foods: Excessive sugar consumption, especially from sugary drinks and highly processed snacks, can contribute to childhood obesity and dental problems. Encouraging children to enjoy sweets in moderation is important.

Portion Control: Teaching children about appropriate portion sizes helps prevent overeating and supports a healthy weight. Understanding portion control also aids in reducing food waste.

Role Modelling: Parents and caregivers play a significant role in shaping children's eating habits through their own behaviour. Being positive role models by consuming a variety of nutritious foods and demonstrating balanced eating habits is essential.

Education: Educating children about nutrition, where food comes from, and the benefits of making healthy choices can empower them to make informed decisions about their diets.

Food Allergies and Dietary Restrictions: Recognizing and accommodating food allergies or dietary restrictions is essential for children's safety and well-being. It's vital for caregivers, schools, and communities to support children with special dietary needs.

School Nutrition Programs: School nutrition programs and cafeteria menus have a substantial impact on children's diets. Efforts to improve the nutritional quality of school meals can significantly contribute to better eating habits among students.

Community Initiatives: Communities can play a role in promoting childhood nutrition through initiatives such as community gardens, farmers' markets, nutrition education programs, and policies that limit the marketing of unhealthy foods to children.

Screen Time and Physical Activity: Balancing screen time with physical activity is essential for overall health. Encouraging children to engage in active play and limit sedentary screen time supports healthy lifestyles.

Topic :13 "School Nutrition Programs" and explore their significance in promoting healthy eating habits among students:

School Meal Programs: School nutrition programs encompass various meal options provided to students during the school day. These typically include breakfast, lunch, and, in some cases, after-school snacks. These programs ensure that students have access to nutritious meals regardless of their family's socioeconomic status.

Nutritional Standards: Many countries have established nutritional standards and guidelines for school meals to ensure they meet specific nutrient and calorie requirements. These standards aim to provide balanced meals that contribute to students' overall health and well-being.

Variety and Balanced Choices: School meal programs often offer a variety of menu options to accommodate different dietary preferences and restrictions. Balanced choices include a combination of fruits, vegetables, lean proteins, whole grains, and low-fat dairy or dairy alternatives.

Reducing Food Insecurity: School meals play a crucial role in addressing food insecurity among students. For many children, school breakfast and lunch may be their most reliable source of nutritious food, especially during weekends and holidays.

Subsidised Meals: In many countries, school meal programs offer subsidised or free meals to students from low-income households. This helps ensure that all students have access to nutritious meals, reducing disparities in food access.

Nutrition Education: Some school meal programs incorporate nutrition education as part of the curriculum. This education can include classroom lessons on healthy eating, understanding food labels, and the importance of a balanced diet.

Dietary Accommodations: School nutrition programs often accommodate students with dietary restrictions or food allergies. Special meals can be provided to ensure these students receive safe and nutritious options.

Promoting Healthy Eating Habits: Exposure to balanced, healthy meals at school can contribute to the development of lifelong healthy eating habits. Students learn about portion control, trying new foods, and the importance of different food groups.

Reducing Junk Food Availability: Some schools have implemented policies to limit the availability of sugary and unhealthy snacks and beverages in vending machines and on campus. This reduces students' access to less nutritious options.

Breakfast Programs: School breakfast programs are particularly important as they provide a nutritious start to the day for students. Research shows that students who eat breakfast are more focused, perform better academically, and have fewer behavioural issues.

Farm-to-School Initiatives: Some school nutrition programs participate in farm-to-school initiatives, where locally sourced foods are incorporated into school meals. This supports local agriculture, reduces food transportation emissions, and provides fresher food options.

Parental and Community Involvement: Engaging parents, caregivers, and the community in school nutrition programs can enhance their success. These stakeholders can provide input, volunteer, and support initiatives that promote healthy eating at school.

Evaluation and Improvement: Regular evaluation of school nutrition programs is essential to ensure they meet nutritional goals and student needs. Feedback from students, parents, and staff can inform improvements and menu adjustments.

Promoting Food Literacy: School meal programs can contribute to food literacy by exposing students to diverse foods, teaching them about food preparation, and encouraging an understanding of where food comes from.

Impact on Health Outcomes: School nutrition programs have the potential to positively impact students' health outcomes by reducing the risk of diet-related health issues, such as obesity, diabetes, and heart disease.

Topic :14 "Mindful Eating" and explore the concept and practices associated with this approach to nutrition:

Definition of Mindful Eating: Mindful eating is an approach to food consumption that emphasises awareness, presence, and a non-judgmental attitude toward eating. It involves paying full attention to the sensory experience of eating, including taste, texture, smell, and even the sounds of food.

Mindfulness Roots: Mindful eating draws inspiration from mindfulness, a meditation practice rooted in Buddhist traditions. It involves being fully present in the moment and cultivating an open, non-reactive awareness.

The Opposite of Mindless Eating: Mindful eating is often contrasted with mindless eating, which involves eating quickly, without awareness, and often in response to external cues like stress or boredom.

Eating with Intention: Mindful eating encourages individuals to eat with intention rather than habit. It involves conscious decision-making about when, what, and how much to eat, rather than responding automatically to cravings or external influences.

Slowing Down: One of the fundamental practices of mindful eating is eating slowly. This allows individuals to savour each bite, fully experience the flavours, and become more attuned to hunger and fullness cues.

Listening to Hunger and Fullness: Mindful eating involves tuning into the body's signals of hunger and fullness. This helps prevent overeating and promotes a more balanced relationship with food.

Non-Judgmental Awareness: Mindful eaters cultivate a non-judgmental attitude toward their eating experiences. They avoid labelling foods as "good" or "bad" and refrain from criticising themselves for their food choices.

Emotional Eating Awareness: Mindful eating encourages individuals to recognize emotional triggers for eating, such as stress, sadness, or boredom. It encourages alternative coping strategies for dealing with emotions.

Mindful Food Choices: When choosing foods, mindful eating involves considering nutritional value, taste preferences, and the body's hunger signals. It discourages restrictive diets or rigid food rules.

Appreciation for Food Sources: Mindful eating fosters an appreciation for the sources of food, including where it comes from, how it's grown, and the efforts involved in its production.

Mindful Meal Planning: Planning meals mindfully involves considering nutritional balance and the satisfaction that different foods provide. It encourages a variety of foods and takes time to enjoy the preparation and consumption of meals.

Reduction of Overeating and Emotional Eating: By increasing awareness of physical hunger and emotional triggers, mindful eating can help individuals reduce episodes of overeating and emotional eating.

Weight Management: Some research suggests that practising mindful eating may be associated with better weight management. It can help individuals become more attuned to their body's natural cues for hunger and fullness.

Stress Reduction: Mindful eating can be a form of stress reduction, as it encourages individuals to eat in a calm and present manner, reducing the tendency to use food as a coping mechanism for stress.

Cultivating Gratitude: Mindful eating often involves pausing to express gratitude for the food and those involved in its production. This practice fosters a deeper connection to food and its origins.

Topic :15 "Nutrition for Seniors" and explore the unique dietary considerations and challenges faced by older adults:

Nutritional Needs in Aging: As individuals age, their nutritional needs change. Seniors require specific nutrients to support healthy ageing, including vitamins, minerals, protein, and fibre.

Caloric Needs: Older adults often require fewer calories than younger individuals due to a decrease in metabolic rate and physical activity. However, nutrient density becomes increasingly important to ensure they meet their nutritional needs without excess calories.

Protein Requirements: Protein is essential for maintaining muscle mass and overall health in seniors. Adequate protein intake helps prevent age-related muscle loss (sarcopenia). Lean meats, poultry, fish, beans, and dairy products are good sources of protein.

Calcium and Vitamin D: Seniors are at greater risk of osteoporosis, so maintaining strong bones is crucial. Calcium and vitamin D intake is important for bone health. Dairy products, leafy greens, and fortified foods are sources of calcium, while sunlight and supplements can provide vitamin D.

Fibre and Digestive Health: Fibre is important for digestive health and can help prevent constipation, a common issue in older adults. Foods like whole grains, fruits, vegetables, and legumes are rich in dietary fibre.

Hydration: Staying hydrated becomes increasingly important as the sense of thirst may diminish with age. Dehydration can lead to health issues, so seniors should aim to drink enough water and consume hydrating foods like fruits and soups.

Micronutrients: Seniors may be at risk of certain micronutrient deficiencies, such as vitamin B12, vitamin B6, and folate. Regular consumption of fortified foods and, if necessary, supplements can help address these deficiencies.

Nutrient Absorption: Aging can affect nutrient absorption in the digestive system. For example, seniors may have reduced absorption of vitamin B12. Healthcare providers may recommend supplements in cases of nutrient malabsorption.

Challenges of Limited Appetite: Some older adults may have a reduced appetite, making it challenging to meet nutritional needs. Providing smaller, nutrient-dense meals and snacks can be a solution.

Oral Health: Dental issues can affect the ability to chew and enjoy a variety of foods. Seniors should practise good oral hygiene and consider softer or more easily chewed foods when necessary.

Social and Psychological Factors: Loneliness, depression, and social isolation can impact dietary habits in older adults. Encouraging social interactions and providing emotional support can positively influence eating habits.

Medication Interactions: Some medications can affect appetite or nutrient absorption. Seniors should discuss potential medication-nutrient interactions with their healthcare providers.

Prevention of Chronic Conditions: A balanced diet rich in fruits, vegetables, whole grains, and lean proteins can help

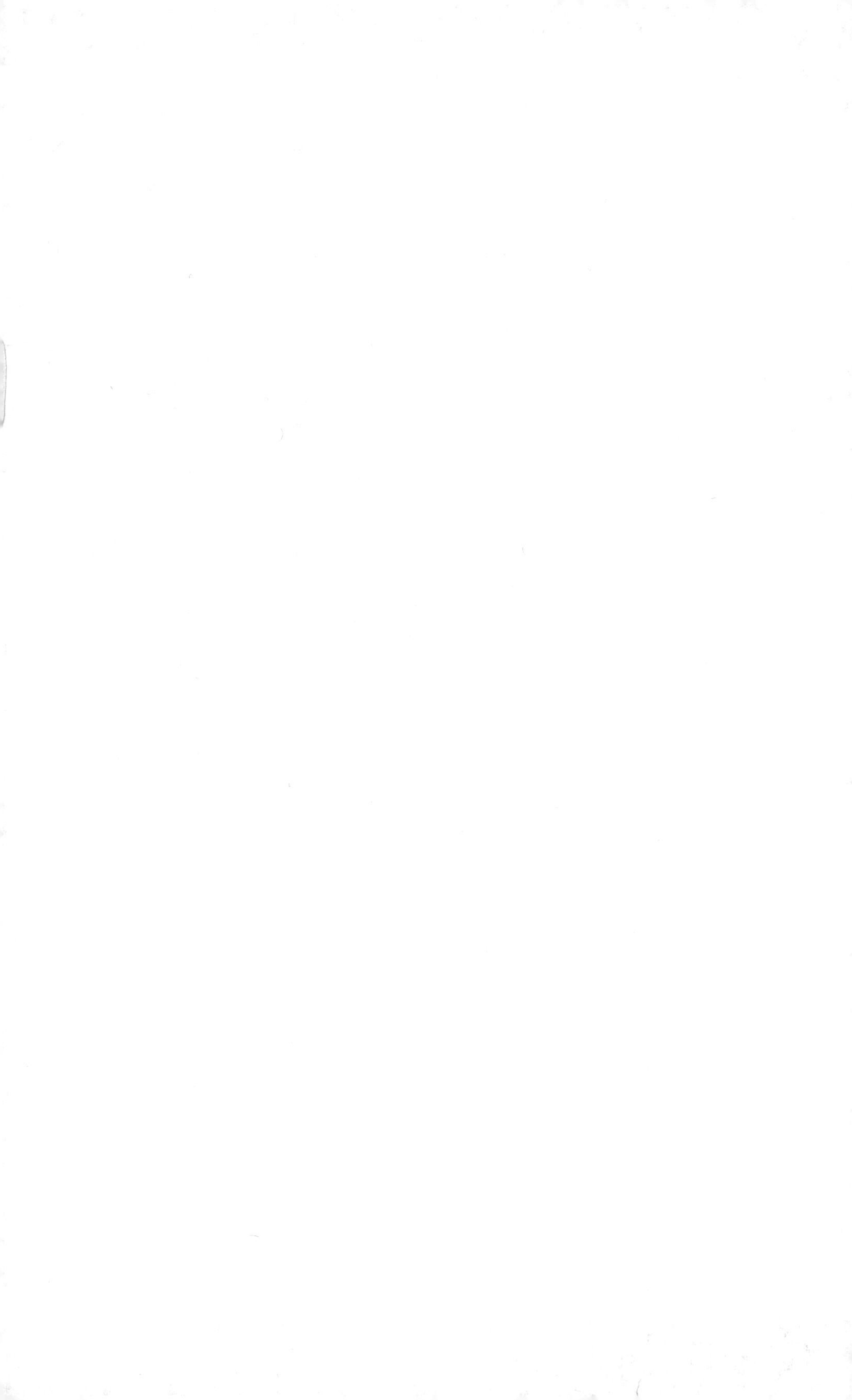